Low Carb Diet

Low Carb Diet Recipes Cookbook for Beginners for Batch Cooking

LELA GIBSON

Introduction

I want to thank you and congratulate you for buying the book, *"Low Carb Diet"*.

This book contains proven steps and strategies on how to prepare low carb meals for batch cooking.

Most people can relate to not feeling like doing much once they get home after a rough day at work. However, imagine having all your meals for the entire week ready. How cool is it getting home after a rough day at work to find ready food and all you need to do is warm the food or just put in the stove for a few minutes and you don't have to wash, cut and prepare the food?

Batching cooking is a very useful method of making meals especially if busy, and who isn't? The most beneficial thing about batch cooking is that you simplify a rather complex and time-consuming process in just a few hours. Batch cooking is especially beneficial when adopting any diet. As you are aware, adopting any new diet is challenging and thus to ensure you stick to the diet and are not tempted to eat what you are not supposed to eat, meal planning is key. Your work is even made easier when you can prepare meals in batch. You not only save time but also save how much of some ingredients you may use.

If you want to learn more about batch cooking especially preparing low carb meals, then this book is perfect for you. In this book, you will learn more about batch cooking as well as some low carb recipes you can prepare in bulk.

Thanks again for buying this book, I hope you enjoy it!

against the publisher for any reparation, damages, or monetary loss due to the information herein, either directly or indirectly.

Respective authors own all copyrights not held by the publisher.

The information herein is offered for informational purposes solely, and is universal as so. The presentation of the information is without contract or any type of guarantee assurance.

The trademarks that are used are without any consent, and the publication of the trademark is without permission or backing by the trademark owner. All trademarks and brands within this book are for clarifying purposes only and are the owned by the owners themselves, not affiliated with this document.

CONTENTS

Introduction   3

1   Batch Cooking In A Nutshell   9

2   Breakfast   12

3   Lunch   21

4   Dinner   33

5   Snacks   49

6   Desserts   55

7   I need your help...   61

8   Preview Of 'Air Fryer Cookbook'   62

9   Bonus: Subscribe To The Free Weight Loss Report   72

Before you learn delicious low carb batch cooking recipes, let's first learn a little bit more about batch cooking.

Batch Cooking In A Nutshell

Batch cooking can be described as planning for or preparing most of your meals or snacks in advance. You can allocate 2-3 hours to make all meals for the entire week in 1 particular day preferably during the weekend. Setting aside a few hours to prep for meals can save time compared to spending up to 60 minutes daily, cooking food for that particular day.

Batch cooking basically takes the mental "burden" off your mind from thinking of what to eat for dinner or if you feel like cooking particularly after a tough day. While eating out could be an option, finding low carb meals can be quite challenging and you are likely not to stick to the diet.

When getting started with batch cooking, it is normal to feel overwhelmed of all the meals to prepare for the entire week but you can simplify things out. One way to make things easier is to begin with particular meals that require prior preparation or if pressed for time with breakfast or dinner, start with that meal and then slowly build upon the days when you can go full throttle! The more you cook in bulk, the better you will become at it. Before you realize it, you'll be a master meal prep machine and time saving guru!

Here's a list of equipment or supplies you may require to make batch cooking easier:

- Several large mixing bowls

- Vitamix or other high-speed blender

- Ziploc sandwich and snack-size bags

- Airtight glass containers or mason jars

- Stove, oven, microwave, instant pot etc

The rule of the thumb with batch cooking is to cook the food "naked", i.e. with no or limited seasonings, no sauces, little or no oil and no dressing at all, and then when it is time to serve, simply reheat the food in a microwave, oven or stove and add various toppings.

You can add dips, sauces, dressings, herbs and fresh seasonings and serve with fresh salad, berries, yoghurt, canned fish or other foods.

Before we look at some recipes you can prepare, below are some tips that will make batch cooking much easier:

Freeze in small portions: It makes no sense to freeze 6 liters of chicken soup for instance unless you are planning to use the soup at once. Freeze according to the portions you will be using during each meal. This makes defrosting much easier.

Get rid of the air: When storing food in a freezer bag, make sure you get rid of the air to prevent freezer burn. You can use a straw to suck out the excess air. If food does not fill a container completely, put a parchment paper over the dish and tuck in the sides to prevent air from getting into the dish.

Label: Make sure you label the different meals you will be freezing. Write what a particular meal is, the quantity, when it was prepared and any recipe directions you may have to know once thawed. This makes cooking much easier and something will not go bad since you know when you prepared it and when it will expire.

Keep track of what you have: Ensure that each week before you prepare the next batch of meals, you know what you have in the freezer. This will ensure that foods don't go bad.

To get started with batch cooking, here are some low carb recipes you can cook in bulk.

Breakfast

Low Carb Breakfast Pockets

Serves 2

Ingredients

1/4 cup shredded cheddar cheese

2 large eggs

1 whole Joseph's Low Carb Lavash

Directions

1. Scramble the eggs and season with your favorite seasonings.

2. To make 4 equal sizes pieces, cut these two halves in half a second time. The pieces should be about 2x4 inches.

3. Now place a pinch of the scrambled eggs and a pinch of cheddar cheese for each of the 4 pieces, and then fold the lavash over the cheddar and eggs.

4. Use a fork to press down the sides to close it (each pocket). Now fry the pockets in oil such as coconut oil for about 10 seconds each side over medium heat.

5. Refrigerate the leftovers for later.

Nutritional Information Per Serving: Calories 197.8, Fat 13.4g, Carbs 8.2g, Protein 14.6g

Mediterranean Eggs

Serves 4

Ingredients

3 ounces feta cheese, crumbled

6-8 large eggs

⅓ cup julienne cut tomatoes, sun dried

1 clove garlic, minced

1 tablespoon extra-virgin olive oil

1 tablespoon butter

1½ large yellow onions, sliced

Ciabatta rolls, if desired

Parsley, finely chopped

Kosher salt, coarse-grained

Black pepper, freshly ground

Directions

1. Heat butter in a stainless steel skillet over medium heat.

2. Once butter has melted, add in the onions and stir and then arrange them in an even layer.

3. Lower the heat for the onions to cook for about 1 hour until they become soft and golden in color. Remember to stir every 5-10 minutes.

4. Add in the sundried tomatoes and garlic and cook for 1-3 minutes while stirring. Cook until fragrant. Transfer this mixture into a container and refrigerate until when you want to eat.

5. To cook the Mediterranean eggs, arrange the mixture in a pan in an even layer. Crack the eggs over the top, sprinkle with salt, pepper and crumbled feta.

6. Use a fitting lid to cover the pan and cook for 10-15 minutes. Closely monitor the egg in the last 3 minutes by jiggling the pan to see if the yolk is done. Cook until the egg yolk doesn't move.

7. Remove from the pan and keep until ready to serve.

8. To serve, sprinkle with chopped parsley and serve on crusty ciabatta rolls.

Nutritional Information Per Serving: Fat 11 g, Carbs 11 g, Protein 9 g

Baked Eggs and Asparagus

Serves 2

Ingredients

1/4 teaspoons black pepper

1/4 teaspoon garlic

2 tablespoons parmesan cheese

4 tablespoons almond meal flour

8 large eggs (whole)

1/2 cup heavy cream

16 spear small asparagus

Directions

1. Preheat the oven to 400 degrees F.

2. Grease an oven safe casserole dish and set it aside.

3. Boil the asparagus spears until tender crisp, in around 2 minutes. Once crisp, drain them and run cold water on them.

3. Pat the asparagus dry and then line them in the greased baking dish. Pour the cream over and crack the eggs over the asparagus.

4. Mix black pepper, garlic, parmesan cheese and the almond

meal in a small bowl.

5. Sprinkle the mixture over the eggs and put in the oven. Cook for around 10 minutes until the yolk is firm, the cream puffs over the edges of the eggs and the topping becomes fragrant and golden brown in color.

6. Divide into two then store in airtight containers in the fridge until when ready to eat.

Nutritional Information Per Serving: Calories 471, Protein 20.8 g, Fat 40.4g, Carbs 10.6g

Breakfast Burrito

Serves 2

Ingredients

4 tablespoons mild chunky salsa

2 low carb tortillas

2 oz. cheddar cheese

4 Eggs

Directions

1. First scramble the eggs, and then sprinkle with shredded cheese on top while still hot. Brown the two sides of the tortillas, and allow to cool.

2. Put the cheese and the eggs at the center of tortilla and wrap tightly, and then put in in the pan and brown the sides.

3. Brown the bottom and top of the tortilla. Remove and transfer to an airtight container and store in the fridge

4. When you want to eat, serve with mild salsa.

Nutritional Information Per Serving: Calories 314.3, Fat 21.4 g, Carbs 12.4 g, Protein 24.5 g

Almond Pancakes with Blueberries

Serves 4

Ingredients

1 cup fresh blueberries

8 tablespoons vanilla whey protein

2 oz. curd creamed cottage cheese

1/4 teaspoons baking powder

1/2 cup dry soy flour, whole grain

3 eggs

1/4 cup blanched almond flour

Directions

1. Mix the baking powder, soy flour, protein powder and almond flour.

2. Stir in the cottage cheese and beaten eggs and continue stirring to blend.

3. Warm a large non-stick skillet over medium heat and use canola oil or butter to lightly grease.

4. Drop the batter onto the skillet, using around 1/4 cup per pancake. After bubbles start to form in each of the pancakes,

flip and then cook the other side until firm. This should be done in around 2 minutes.

5. Store the pancakes in a container and serve with the blueberries when you want to eat.

Nutritional Information Per Serving: Calories 212, Carbs 11.3 g, Protein 20.3 g, Fat 10 g

Lunch

Grilled Lamb Chops and Chimichurri

Serves 4

Ingredients

8 (4 oz.) lamb loin chops, trimmed

1/2 teaspoon black pepper, freshly ground

3/4 teaspoon kosher salt, divided

2 garlic cloves, minced

1/8 teaspoon red pepper, crushed

2 teaspoons shallots, minced

1 1/2 tablespoons white vinegar

2 tablespoons low-sodium chicken broth

2 1/2 tablespoons extra-virgin olive oil

1/2 cup fresh flat-leaf parsley

1 1/2 cups fresh mint

Cooking spray

Directions

1. In a food processor, mix ¼ teaspoon pepper, ¼ teaspoon salt, red pepper, shallots, vinegar, broth, oil, parsley and mint.

2. Process the ingredients until fully incorporated.

3. Season the lamb chops with remaining salt and pepper on both sides.

4. Heat a grill pan over medium heat and then use cooking spray to coat the pan.

5. Add the lamb to the pan and cook for 5 minutes on both sides for around 5 minutes each.

6. Store the lamb chops and sauce in separate containers.

Nutritional Information Per Serving: Calories 303 Fat 18.4 g Protein 30.1 g Carbs 4.4 g

Pork Meatballs

Yields 30

Ingredients

1 lb. ground pork

1 tablespoon beef stock

1/2 teaspoon salt

1 large egg, slightly beaten

1 tablespoon less sodium soy sauce

1 tablespoon sriracha chili sauce

1/3 cup panko crispy plain bread crumbs

Directions

1. Preheat the oven to about 375 degrees F. Use a foil to line a baking sheet and then spray it with cooking spray.

2. Mix the ground pork, beef stock, salt, slightly beaten egg, sodium soy sauce, sriracha chili sauce and crispy bread crumbs in a mixing bowl.

3. Shape the mixture into 30 one-inch balls and put in a pan.

4. Bake the meatballs for about 25-30 minutes. To know if the meatballs are ready, they should not be pink in the

center.

5. Freeze the meatballs until when ready to use.

Nutritional Information Per Meatball: Calories 241, Carb 6.24g, Protein 14.74g, Fat 17.10g

Cream Cheese Stuffed Meatballs

Yields 25

Ingredients

3 tablespoons finely diced sun-dried tomatoes

2 slices finely chopped bacon

1 slightly beaten egg

Salt and pepper to taste

750g ground pork

1 clove garlic crushed

1 finely sliced spring onion

2 tablespoons rosemary, thyme, oregano and sage

For filling

110g cream cheese, diced

Directions

1. To make the meatballs, put the ingredients in a mixing bowl then combine with your hands.

2. Scoop a golf-size of the meatball mixture using a dessertspoon. Squeeze the mixture to form a ball, and then flatten the ball into a circle.

3. To make the filling, put a cube of cream cheese in the meatball at the center.

4. Close meatball mixture around the cheese and put the cream cheese stuffed balls on a greased baking tray.

5. Repeat until you've used all the mixture and then spray them with olive oil cooking spray. This helps to make them crisp and brown properly.

6. Bake at 350 degrees F until golden brown, say for around 15 to 20 minutes.

Nutritional Information Per Meatball: Calories 103, Fat 7.5 g Carbohydrates 0.7 g Protein 7.8 g

Chicken Legs & Brussels Sprouts

Serves 2

Ingredients

1/4 cup chicken stock

Juice of 1 lemon

1 tablespoon olive oil, for sprouts

Salt and pepper

Granulated garlic

1 tablespoon of coconut oil

1 stalk of Brussels sprouts, stemmed and chopped

2 whole chicken legs, with skin on & bone

Parmesan cheese to garnish

Directions

1. Preheat the oven to 425 degrees F as you prepare and de-stem the Brussels sprouts.

2. Toss the Brussels sprouts into the olive oil, and season with granulated garlic, salt and pepper.

3. Wash the chicken legs and pat them dry; and then season the chicken with granulated garlic, salt and pepper. Set it

aside.

4. Heat coconut oil in a cast iron, until a drop of water added to the oil produces a hissing and sizzling sound.

5. Add the chicken legs to the pan face down and let it sit for 6-8 minutes to get crispy. Do not move it before it has crisped up.

6. Once done, flip the chicken leg and then allow the other side to crisp too. Wait for some time then add in the Brussels sprouts to the pan together with lemon juice and chicken broth, and stir.

7. Put the contents of the pan into a Ziploc bag until when you want to eat.

8. Place the pan in the oven to bake until the juices run clear and the chicken is well cooked through. This should take about 30 minutes.

9. Garnish with freshly grated cheese and then serve. Cheese makes the dish super tasty!

Nutritional Information Per Serving: Calories 267.2, Fat 15.1 g, Carbs 4.0g, Protein 28.3g

Salmon Quiche

Serves 10

Ingredients

250 ml full fat milk or cream

250g cream cheese diced/cubed

8 eggs

500g salmon fillet, diced/cubed

1 teaspoon dried dill

Pinch of salt and pepper

Directions

1. Whisk the eggs and season with pepper and salt. Add in the milk and mix.

2. Add in cream cheese and diced salmon, and mix gently using a fork.

3. Pour the mixture into a greased dish. Move the pieces of the fish around to distribute them evenly.

4. Bake the contents at 350 degrees F for about 30 minutes.

5. If need be, make the egg mixture and put in a tin, then add salmon pieces evenly to avoid any clumping together.

6. Serve and store the leftovers in airtight containers and refrigerate.

Nutritional Information Per Serving: Calories 207 Fat 16.2 g Carbs 2.2 g Protein 17.2 g

Tomato & Feta Meatballs

Yields 16

Ingredients

Olive oil for frying

2 tablespoons water

1/4 cup almond flour

1/2 teaspoon garlic powder

1 egg

1/2 teaspoon dried thyme or 1 tablespoon fresh thyme leaves

2 tablespoons sundried tomatoes, chopped

1/4 cup crumbled feta cheese

1 lb. ground turkey

Directions

1. In a medium bowl, mix the water, almond flour, garlic powder, egg, thyme, tomatoes and ground turkey.

2. From this mixture, make about 16-inch meatballs and fry in olive oil, in a large sauté pan.

3. Cook the meatballs for around 3-4 minutes, and turn them over.

4. Cook again for 3-4 minutes up until the outsides brown and are well cooked.

5. Remove from the pan and transfer onto a plate lined with paper towel to absorb the extra oil.

6. Once done, you can refrigerate until ready to serve.

7. You can eat the meatballs on their own or serve with spaghetti squash and vegetables to make a full meal.

Nutritional Information Per Meatball: Calories 89, Fat 8g, Carbs 0.65g, Protein 6g

Dinner

Low Carb Shepherd's Pie

Serves 8

Ingredients

3 carrots grated/shredded

60 ml beef stock

400g tinned/canned chopped tomatoes

2 cloves garlic crushed

500g ground lamb or beef

1 red onion diced

Extra virgin olive oil

Cauliflower Mash Topping

50g grated/shredded cheese

Salt and pepper to taste

30ml double/heavy cream

1 small cauliflower cut into pieces

55 g butter

Directions

1. Heat olive oil in a saucepan then fry the garlic and red onion until cooked. Do not brown the ingredients.

2. Add the ground meat and stir until the mixture is browned and cooked.

3. Now add the beef stock, grated carrots and chopped tomatoes and mix.

4. Lower the heat and let it simmer for about 10 minutes, uncovered as you prepare the cauliflower topping. Allow the liquid to evaporate so that the mince can thicken.

Cauliflower Topping

1. Simply boil the cauliflower for about 8 to 10 minutes, or until soft.

2. Drain and let all the steam escape as excess water in the saucepan can make the mash "sloppy".

3. Add the cream, pepper, salt and butter. Puree the mixture using a stick blender that has a blade attachment.

4. To assemble the meal, put the pie in the bottom of a big casserole dish and top with the cauliflower mash. Sprinkle with grated or shredded cheese.

5. Put the dish on a baking tray to any liquids that may

bubble over.

6. Bake at 350 degrees F until the cheese is browned, say for around 20 minutes. Keep refrigerated or store in an airtight glass container until ready to serve.

Nutritional Information Per Serving: Calories 284, Fat 18.5 g, Carbs 10g, Protein 20g

Chicken Teriyaki

Serves 2

Ingredients

10 drops liquid sweetener

Pepper to taste

1 tablespoon ginger powder

1 tablespoon garlic powder

1 tablespoon white vinegar

3 tablespoons olive oil

1 tablespoon Worcestershire sauce

7 tablespoons soy sauce

600g chicken breast, skinned and boned

Directions

1. Mix soy sauce, pepper, ginger, sweetener, garlic, vinegar, Worcestershire sauce and olive oil in a bowl to make the marinade.

2. Dice your chicken and then put into the container with the marinade and put in the fridge for at least 30 minutes to marinate.

3. Cook the chicken in the frying pan over medium heat.

4. Cook until there is no longer any liquid and then keep refrigerated until ready to serve.

Nutritional Information Per Serving: Calories 620, Fat 23g, Protein 90g, Carbs 4g

Zucchini Noodles

Serves 4

Ingredients

2-3 tablespoons prepared basil pesto

2 cups broccoli florets

1/2 cup green onions cut into 1-inch pieces

6 slices of uncooked bacon

Generous pinch of salt

4 medium zucchini, julienned thinly

Romano or Parmesan cheese, for garnish

Directions

1. Put the zucchini in a colander in the sink or over a bowl and then sprinkle with salt. Toss to combine.

2. Let the zucchini sit for about 15 minutes then drain the excess water by squeezing the zucchini.

3. Cook the bacon in a skillet over medium heat, until crisp, as you turn it regularly. Once cooked, put the bacon onto paper towels to dry.

4. Crumble the bacon and remove the bacon drippings; but

reserve about 2 tablespoons of the drippings.

5. Return the pan to heat and add in broccoli and green onions. Stir frequently and cook over medium heat until crisp tender, in about 3-5 minutes.

6. Add in 2 tablespoons of pesto and zucchini and toss to combine. Taste and adjust the seasonings as desired and let it warm up for 2-3 minutes.

7. Store the zucchini noodles and bacon crumbles in separate Ziploc bags. When serving, serve the zucchini noodles with freshly grated Parmesan cheese and bacon crumbles.

Nutritional Information Per Serving: Calories 107.0, Fat 5.1g, Carbs 3.6g, Protein 10.3g

Low Carb Pot Roast

Serves 10

Ingredients

2 tablespoons apple cider vinegar

1/2 teaspoon black pepper

1 tablespoon chili powder

1 teaspoon dried oregano

1 tablespoon coriander, ground

2 tablespoons cumin, ground

1 teaspoon salt

1/2 cup red and yellow peppers cut into strips

1 teaspoon garlic powder

2 tablespoons dried onion flakes

1 cup diced tomatoes

1/2 cup canned green chilies, chopped

1/2 cup salsa Verde

2.5 – 3 lbs. boneless chuck roast

Directions

1. Season the roast with sufficient amount of salt and pepper and then sear in a hot pan until browned on all sides. Position the roast in a 5-quart slow cooker.

2. Add the tomatoes, chilies and salsa Verde to the pan that you used to sear the meat. Deglaze and bring the mixture to a boil.

3. Pour the mixture over the meat in the slow cooker and add in apple cider vinegar, black pepper, chili powder, oregano, coriander, cumin, salt, peppers, garlic and onion flakes.

4. Cook the contents on high for about 4 hours or until the meat is tender.

5. Once done, shred it. Serve with preferred topping and refrigerate the leftovers.

Nutritional Information Per Serving: Calories 271, Fat 19g, Carbs 2g, Protein 20g

Low Carb Meatloaf

Serves 12

Ingredients

6 slices bacon to cover the meatloaf

Diced/grated/shredded vegetables

2 teaspoons dried oregano

2 tablespoons chopped sun-dried tomatoes

2 slices bacon, diced

Handful fresh basil, chopped

Handful fresh parsley, chopped

2 lightly beaten eggs

750g ground pork

750g ground beef

2 cloves garlic crushed

1 spring onion sliced

Salt and pepper to taste

3.5 grated cheese, optional

Directions

1. Grease and line a baking dish and set aside. Add all ingredients to a mixing bowl then mix using your hands to fully incorporate them.

2. Make a large meatloaf and put on the prepared baking tray. Cover with bacon slices then sprinkle with cheese if you like.

3. Bake at 350 degrees F until well cooked in the center, say in 50 minutes or so.

4. Store in an airtight container until when ready to eat.

Nutritional Information Per Serving: Calories 370 Fat 25 g Carbs 1.2 g Protein 35 g

Crockpot Bulgur

Serves 6

Ingredients

1 tablespoon lemon peel, finely shredded

1/3 cup fresh mint or cilantro, chopped

1/4 teaspoon salt

1 tablespoon fresh ginger, grated

1 tablespoon canola oil

1 medium jalapeno Chile pepper, sliced

1 1/2 cups water

3/4 cup bulgur, rinsed and drained

Nonstick cooking spray

Lemon wedges, optional

Jalapeno Chile pepper slices, optional

Directions

1. Using the cooking spray, lightly coat your slow cooker then add in bulgur, salt, ginger, oil, sliced jalapeno and water.

2. Cook the mixture on low heat for about 1 ½ hours then

stir in lemon peel and mint.

3. Serve the bulgur at room temperature and garnish with lemon wedges and jalapeno slices. Store the leftovers.

Nutritional Information Per Serving: Calories 83, Carbs 14 g, Fat 3g, protein 2g

Thai-style fish cakes

Serves 4

Ingredients

1/3 cup vegetable oil

50g green beans, finely chopped

3 green shallots, finely chopped

1 egg, lightly whisked

2 tablespoons sweet chili sauce

2 tablespoons fish sauce

1/4 cup corn-flour

1/2 cup fresh coriander leaves

500 g firm white fish fillets, coarsely chopped

Sweet chili sauce, extra

Lime wedges, to serve

For Herb & peanut salad

2 teaspoons fresh lime juice

2 tablespoons olive oil

2 tablespoons roasted peanuts, chopped

1/2 cup fresh coriander leaves

50g Asian salad mix

Directions

1. Place the firm white fish fillets in a food processor, and process until it's smooth.

2. Add in the egg, sweet chili sauce, fish sauce, corn flour and coriander, and continue to process until fully combined.

3. Pour the mixture into a larger bowl, and then add in the beans and shallot, and stir to combine.

4. Heat some oil in a frying pan over medium heat, and then put 4 egg rings in the hot pan.

5. Sub-divide the fish mixture into eight portions, and press one portion into each of the egg ring.

6. Cook the mixture for around 4 minutes each side or until golden brown.

7. Transfer the fish cakes to a plate with paper towel and do the same with the remaining mixture.

8. You can freeze the fish cakes until when you want to eat.

9. When you want to serve, prepare the salad by combining lime juice, oil, peanuts, coriander and Asian salad mix in a large bowl.

10. Divide the salad and the fish cakes amongst the serving plates and then serve over extra sweet chili sauce and lime wedges.

Nutritional Information Per Serving: Calories 500, fat 35 g, protein 35 g, Carbs 12 g

Snacks

Baked Parmesan

Serves 12

Ingredients

12 heaped tablespoons grated parmesan

Optional: poppy and/or sesame seeds

Directions

1. Preheat the oven to around 400 degrees F. Meanwhile, lay a baking sheet in a tray.

2. Pick a big cookie cutter that has a simple circular shape but with no bottom.

3. Press the cutter into the sheet and spread a heaped tablespoon of parmesan into the cutter as evenly as possible.

4. Use your fingers to press the cheese, and ensure it remains regularly spread.

5. Lift your cutter and continue with this process to make the number of crackers you want.

6. Bake the crackers for around 10 minutes, until the cheese starts to melt. As the parmesan may start to burn within a few seconds, pay close attention.

7. When serving, you can incorporate a little sesame or poppy seeds in order to improve the flavor.

8. The baked parmesan freezes really well.

Nutritional Information Per Serving: Calories 22, Fat 1 g, Protein 2 g, carb 0 g

Zucchini Crisps

Serves 4

Ingredients

1 teaspoon thyme

¼ teaspoon black pepper, ground

1 teaspoon garlic powder

1 teaspoon sea salt

1 egg

1 cup almond flour

1 large zucchini, sliced into rings

Directions

1. Preheat the oven to 450 degrees F and then position a rack in the middle of the oven.

2. Use parchment paper to line a baking sheet and set it aside.

3. Lightly beat the egg in a small bowl, and then mix black pepper, thyme, garlic powder, salt and almond flour in a separate bowl.

4. Now insert the zucchini slices into the egg and allow the

excess to fall off, and then put into the almond flour mix bowl and coat.

5. Position the coated slices of zucchini onto the lined baking sheet.

6. Bake for about 6 minutes on every side. Store the crisps in a Ziploc bag and store in the refrigerator. You can serve with any low carb sauce you like.

Nutritional Information Per Serving: Calories 112, Fat 9g, Carbs 6g, Protein 6 g

Fried Cheddar

Serves 1

Ingredients

2 tablespoons olive oil

2 teaspoons hemp nuts

2 teaspoons almond flour

2 teaspoons ground flaxseed

2 eggs

4 slices cheddar, 50 grams each

Salt and pepper to taste

Directions

1. Heat a tablespoon of olive oil in a frying pan, over medium heat. Meanwhile whisk the egg, pepper and salt together in a separate bowl.

2. Combine almond flour with ground flaxseed and the hemp nuts.

3. Use the egg mix to coat the cheddar slices, and then with the hemp nut mix.

4. Fry the cheese slices for around 3 minutes on each side.

Store until ready to eat, and serve it while hot.

Nutritional Information Per Serving: Calories 588, Fat 48g, Protein 35g Carbs 5g

Desserts

Coconut Fluff

Serves 2

Ingredients

2 teaspoons SF vanilla flavoring syrup

2 tablespoons heavy whipping cream

2 oz. cream cheese

2 tablespoons coconut spread

2 tablespoons coconut flakes, unsweetened

Directions

1. Toast your coconut flakes lightly and then stir in the coconut spread/butter, heating the mixture for about 30 seconds.

2. Stir in the cubed and softened cream cheese and microwave for around 30 seconds. Continue to stir to obtain a soft and airy mixture.

3. Add in the flavoring syrup and whipping cream, and stir to fully blend.

4. Keep in the fridge or freezer to firm up. Serve this as a

whipped dessert after it has cooled. You can also keep in the fridge until when ready to eat.

Nutritional Information Per Serving: Calories 321.8, Fat 32.6g, Carbs 6.4g, Protein 3.3g

Ricotta Cheese with Vanilla

Serves 2

Ingredients

2 tablespoons Crème fraîche

2 sachets vanilla flavoring

400g Ricotta cheese, 2% fat

Directions

1. Combine the crème fraiche with the ricotta cheese and then add in the vanilla sachet.

2. If you want to make your homemade vanilla flavoring, just scrape vanilla pod's pulp and then mix it with a little liquid sweetener.

3. Refrigerate until when ready to eat.

Nutritional Information Per Serving: Calories 290, Fat 18 g, Protein 8 g, Carbs 3 g

Berries with Chocolate Ganache

Serves 6

Ingredients

8 oz. strawberries

2 cups red raspberries

2 cups fresh blueberries

8 ounce chocolate chips, sugar free

1/3 cup heavy cream

1/2 teaspoon vanilla extract

Directions

1. Mix the fruits and put in dessert bowls.

2. Heat the cream and chocolate over low heat until melted, or alternatively microwave for around 30 seconds.

3. Add the vanilla and stir to get a smooth consistency.

4. Cool slightly and pour the chocolate over the fruits and serve; this desert freezes well.

Nutritional Information Per Serving: Calories 260, Protein 2.3g, Fat 17.8g, Carbs 19.1g

Cheesecake Cups

Servings: 12

Ingredients

2 large eggs

1 teaspoon vanilla extract

1/2 cup xylitol

12 oz. cream cheese

Directions

1. Preheat your oven to about 350 degrees F.

2. Use a non-stick cooking spray to coat a 12-cup muffin tin. Mix xylitol and cream cheese using a mixer until creamy.

3. Now add in eggs and vanilla extract one at a time and mix. Add in equal proportions into the 12 cup muffin tin.

4. Bake for about 40 minutes and then allow to cool. Refrigerate the egg cups in Ziploc bags until when ready to serve.

5. When serving, fill the cake with mixed berries and top with whipped topping.

Chocolate Cake

Serves 2

Ingredients

1/2 teaspoon baking powder

4 teaspoons sucralose based sweetener

2 cups liquid egg whites

1.4 oz. dark chocolate

1 cup chocolate almond milk, unsweetened

4 scoops chocolate protein powder

4 tablespoons cocoa powder, unsweetened

Directions

1. In a mixing bowl, mix baking powder, the sweetener, egg whites, dark chocolate, almond milk, protein powder and cocoa powder.

2. Pour the batter into a cake pan and bake in a preheated oven at 375 degrees F for around 25 minutes.

3. Serve or store to snack on a few days later.

Nutritional Information Per Serving: Calories 73, Carb 3.10g, Proteins 10.01g, Fat 2.15g

I need your help...

Thank you again for downloading this book!

I hope this book was able to help you to get low carb recipes.

The next step is to take action and follow the low carb diet.

Finally, if you enjoyed this book, would you be kind enough to leave a review for this book on Amazon?

I want to reach as many people as I can with this book, and more reviews will help me accomplish that!

If you have any questions or problems, please contact us: hello@freedomdestination.com

Thank you and good luck!

Preview Of 'Air Fryer Cookbook'

Firstly, you need to appreciate that despite the name, no frying happens in this appliance. Since the common understanding of frying usually means to cook in fat, the air fryer does not do that.

The Air fryer is a countertop convection oven (meaning it is an oven with a fan inside) that is self-contained and has a vertical orientation—the fan located at the top blows down through an electric heating component. The airflow begins at the top, heats up, and then moves fast around your food through a netting-cooking basket, and then down to a shaped drip tray that circulates the air back to the top. To use the device, you position the food you intend to 'fry' at the center of this airflow.

The mesh basket, so you know, resembles a deep fry basket. In this appliance, you will not find an oil reservoir or anything like it.

The General Features and Benefits of the Air Fryer

The air fryer has the following features and benefits:

Promotes low fat

First, you don't even have to add any oil when you are air-frying frozen food that is meant to be used for baking. You only need to take the food from the freezer, place it directly into the air fryer, and then set the temperature and timer. For raw meat, you also do not require any oil; the quick circulating hot air will cook your meat at all angles to give your meat a crispy outside and a moist inside. The excess fat from the meat will drip down the tray right below the cooking basket.

With the air fryer, you can try fried chicken wings, meat patties, pork chops, hot air dried fish, roast chicken, crackling roast pork, steaks, and all other meat dishes you love.

It's automatic

While using the air fryer, the cooking process is a simple one. We have two popular types of hot fryers on retail: the paddle Tefal Actifry, and the mesh bottom-cooking basket that sits on a drip tray.

The former is the only one that comes with a stirring paddle; the other hot fryer brands in the market use the cooking basket design. You may also have noted that these hot fryers usually have their own air fryer accessories.

When using the Tefal Actifry air fryer, the only thing you have to do is place the chopped ingredients inside the cooking bowl. The machine will do the entire cooking process for you; the stirring paddle stirs the food gently as the bowl rotates. This definitely frees up your time for other things like making some salad to go with your food. Otherwise, you can just sit there and wait for the timer to beep when the food is ready.

NOTE: For the basket-style air fryer, you may need to shake the tinier cuts or flip the larger cuts over halfway through the cooking.

This machine is therefore incomparable with the hob cooking or the traditional stove that forces you to stand in front of the hot stove for the entire cooking process.

Imagine you are rushing to work in the morning; the last thing you want is to start cleaning up the usual mess after preparing breakfast. The hands-free and quick cooking quality the air fryer brings makes it win over the frying pan or skillet.

It's fuss-free

The air fryer only has 2 buttons, thus making it easy to use the air fryer. By adjusting the temperature and the timer, the meal will be ready when the timer goes off.

The Tefal Actifry makes things even easier because it only has the timer: the temperature setting is fixed. While hot air cookers usually come with pre-set programs, if you are unsure of the right temperature or cooking time, you can press the button for the type of food you are cooking. For instance, if you are cooking chicken, you just press the chicken icon button. The shortcut starter buttons takes out the guesswork out of air frying: fuss-free and simple!

Quick and convenient

You do not need to preheat the compact air fryer before you start cooking. You can easily transfer your frozen French Fries, nuggets, potato wedges and other ingredients directly into the fryer. Adjust the timer and temperature and a few minutes later, beep! Your food is ready.

Perhaps you feel like eating some roasted walnuts or groundnuts while watching football. That is no longer a big deal. Just wash them, place them in the air fryer, and wait to hear the beep.

Additionally, crispy food remains crispy when you reheat it. I do not know about you but I think this is better than buying fat and salt laden food at the fast food joints.

Finally, when cooking smaller food portions, you will find this gadget more practical than the ordinary convection oven. The fryer cooks faster and is economical too (concerning time and fuel consumption).

It's a multi-cooker

A machine that bakes, fries, grills, and roasts is undeniably a highly versatile appliance. Think about it; you have a deep fryer, toaster, skillet, hot grill, and an oven all fitted into one machine! You can use the air fryer for lunch, breakfast, and dinner to make sandwiches, grilled pork chop for dinner, and even snacks for lunch.

As you already know, we are living in a fast-paced world. The extremely versatile hot air fryer brings simplicity, ease, convenience, and so much more to your cooking process; if you do not like cooking, the air fryer's inventor must have had you in mind when inventing the device!

It's easy to clean

The best part is that all the air cooker's removable parts are dishwasher-safe. If you do not own a dishwasher, just soaking and gentle rubbing the parts with a clean sponge is good enough to get rid of all the bits of food stuck on the cooking surface.

Moreover, the appliance comes with a cover and you do all the cooking inside the machine. Unlike the oven or deep fryer, skillet or frying pan that all have an exposed cooking surface, with the air fryer, you will not find oil vapors deposited on your counter top, floor, or walls. This means the only thing that requires cleaning is the drip pan and cooking basket.

It is a food separator and food filter

Some cool air fryers available in the market today have a food separator that lets you cook multiple foods at the same time. For instance, if you want to prepare frozen chicken nuggets and French fries, you can use a separator to prepare the two simultaneously and while doing so, keep the flavors from mixing.

The air fryers also come with an air filter that ensures all the unwanted food odors and vapors do not spread around the house. Once you start using this device, you will have no more wafting food smells coming from your house since the air filter diffuses the hot air steam that floats and sticks. You will thus be able to enjoy your fresh kitchen smell before you start cooking, when you are cooking, and even after cooking.

So how exactly can an air fryer help you to become healthier? That's what we will discuss next.

Check out the rest of Air Fryer Cookbook: Quick, Healthy and Easy Low Carb Air Fryer Recipes on Amazon.

Or go to: http://amzn.to/2icNEqE

Check Out My Other Books

Below you'll find some of my other popular books that are popular on Amazon and Kindle as well. Simply search for these titles on the Amazon website to find them. Alternatively, you can visit my author page on Amazon to see other work done by me.

Instant Pot: Instant Pot Pressure Cooker Cookbook With Easy And Healthy Recipes

Dash Diet: Cookbook for Weight Loss with Action Plan and Easy Recipes

Slow Cooker: Cookbook With Slow Cooker Recipes

Anti-Inflammatory Diet Guide: The Guide to Reduce Inflammation and Live A Healthy Life Without Pain

Negative Calorie Diet: Cookbook & Guide Which Will Help You to Burn Body Fat, Lose Weight and Live Healthy

Anti-Inflammatory Diet Guide: The Guide to Reduce Inflammation and Live a Healthy Life Without Pain

Negative Calorie Diet & Dash Diet Box Set

Negative Calorie Diet & Weight Loss Box Set

Intermittent Fasting: The Essential Beginners Guide for Women for Weight Loss

Negative Calorie Diet & Anti-Inflammatory Diet Guide Box Set

Slow Cooker & Instant Pot Box Set

Negative Calorie Diet & Clean Eating Box Set

Leptin Resistance: Leptin Diet to Control Your Hormones, Get Permanent Weight Loss, Cure Obesity and Live Healthy

Weight Loss: 20 Easy and Fast Diet Tips for Losing Weight – an Easy-to-Follow Weight Loss Guide

Belly Diet: The Zero Belly Diet Step-by-Step Guide Which Helps You To Lose Your Belly and Enjoy Your Flat Belly

Belly Diet Smoothies: Delicious Smoothie Recipes to Flatten Your Belly, Improve Your Gut & Burn Fat

Weight Loss Cookbook: Meal Prep Cookbook For Weight Loss and Clean Eating

Smart Fat: Cookbook with Fat Meals Which Help You to Lose Weight, Get Healthy and Improve Brain Function

Clean Eating: Cookbook and Guide to Restore Your Body's Natural Balance and Eat Healthy

Negative Calorie Diet & Smart Fat Box Set

Weight Loss: 20 Easy and Fast Diet Tips for Losing Weight – an Easy-to-Follow Weight Loss Guide

Paleo Smoothies: Recipes to Energize and for Ultimate Health and Weight Loss

Ketogenic Cookbook: Quick Low Calorie Ketogenic Crockpot Recipes with 7 Days Meal Plan

Air Fryer Cookbook: Quick, Healthy and Easy Low Carb Air Fryer Recipes

Bonus: Subscribe To The Free Weight Loss Report

When you subscribe to Freedom Destination via email, you will get free access to an ebook. All you have to do is enter your email address to get instant access.

The Introduction Manual is more than just an introduction to the diet. Instead, it discusses the science behind how we gain and lose weight as well as what absolutely needs to be done to attack that stubborn body fat that, until now, has been so challenging to get rid of.

Here are the preview of what you'll get:

- Rapid Weight Loss

- How This System Works

- Why This Diet

- Why 3 Weeks?

- 21 Days To Make A Habit

- Fat Loss VS. Weight Loss

- Nutrients

- Protein, Fat, Carbohydrates

- The Food Pyramid And Obesity

- Fiber

- Metabolism

- How We Get Fat

- Triglycerides

- How To Get Thin

- Diet Overview

- Meal Frequency

- Water

- Diet Essentials

- Let's Get Started

You can access it here: http://bit.ly/2tUb9cp